Best Ab
Exercises

**Abdominal Workout Routine
For Core Strength And A Flat
Stomach**

Patrick Barrett

CONTENTS

"There are rich rewards in developing a trim mid-section. All your internal organs receive benefit."

-Cpl. Marvin Urvant, Strength and Health magazine, April 1945

Books by Patrick Barrett:

Natural Exercise: Basic Bodyweight Training and Calisthenics for Strength and Weight-Loss

The Natural Diet: Simple Nutritional Advice For Optimal Health In The Modern World

How To Do A Handstand: From the Basic Exercises To The Free Standing Handstand Pushup

Best Ab Exercises: Abdominal Workout Routine For Core Strength And A Flat Stomach

Hand And Forearm Exercises: Grip Strength Workout And Training Routine

Advanced Bodyweight Exercises: An Intense Full Body Workout In A Home Or Gym

One Arm Pull Up: Bodyweight Training And Exercise Program For One Arm Pull Ups And Chin Ups

Easy Exercises: Simple Workout Routine For Busy People In The Office, At Home, Or On The Road

Disclaimer:

INTRODUCTION

Hi. My name is Patrick Barrett, and I'd like to thank you for buying this book.

Core strength—strength throughout your abdomen, lower back, and the side muscles between them—is an essential component of your overall strength and health. Many people think of ab exercises as essentially cosmetic, because their goals are more associated with having an attractive looking stomach over a flabby one.

There's nothing wrong with having that goal, especially if it drives you to eat better and work out your core, and this book will help you to make that goal a reality.

But this book will also go beyond that, because exercising your abs and your lower back is important for bigger reasons than the cosmetic ones. If you go about it in the right way, you can build very real strength that translates well to the real world, and you can lay the necessary foundation for avoiding potential back pain and general discomfort that many people experience as they age.

In this book, you'll learn everything that you need to build an attractive mid-section. Even more importantly, you'll be able to develop real strength in your core, which can pay off for a long time in a lot of ways you might not even be aware of.

But, as always, this information will only help you if you put it to work. Everything we just talked about depends on you finishing this book and applying what you learned.

So let's go ahead and get started—the faster we get into it, the faster you can start making progress.

Other Books by Patrick Barrett:

Natural Exercise*: Basic Bodyweight Training and Calisthenics for Strength and Weight-Loss*

The Natural Diet*: Simple Nutritional Advice For Optimal Health In The Modern World*

How To Do A Handstand*: From the Basic Exercises To The Free Standing Handstand Pushup*

One Arm Pull Up*: Bodyweight Training And Exercise Program For One Arm Pull Ups And Chin Ups*

Advanced Bodyweight Exercises*: An Intense Full Body Workout In A Home Or Gym*

Easy Exercises*: Simple Workout Routine For Busy People In The Office, At Home, Or On The Road*

Hand And Forearm Exercises*: Grip Strength Workout And Training Routine*

THE BEST KIND OF AB ROUTINE

Perhaps more than ever, people are very, very conscious about their midsections.

People of all ages want to keep their stomachs trim and attractive, and they buy all kinds of in-home gadgets, not to mention gym memberships, DVDs, and, yes, exercise books, in the hopes of reaching that goal.

I can understand the importance of having an attractive physique, and you can certainly make that happen with the exercises in this book.

But beside their cosmetic function, your abdominal muscles and lower back are enormously important in the context of your overall physical strength.

Strength is obviously important for athletes, but even outside of an athletic context, the strength in your core—abs and lower back—is a huge part of what regulates your posture and what keeps you from having back problems and other similar issues as you age.

So you want an ab workout routine with ab exercises that fulfill the cosmetic need, but also give you real strength that your body can use in the sports arena tomorrow as well as for just "getting around" as you get older.

That means you need exercises that work out your core in conjunction with the rest of your body, and this is where a lot of mainstream abdominal workouts fall short—they primarily employ exercises that focus on your stomach without engaging the rest of your body at the same time.

That can cause problems for you, because it's not how things happen in real life.

In most situations, your stomach and lower back create stability for the rest of your body so that it can do what it does in a better, more stable environment. In these real life instances, your core works with the rest of your body at the same time—which is why in your workouts, your core should work simultaneously with your body, not in isolation from it.

You want ab exercises that focus on your stomach, but they should also engage other major muscle groups as well.

This makes sure that not only do you have that attractive, strong physique that you want, but when you leave the gym you can actually use all of those muscles you've been building without hurting yourself—and decades down the road they're still working for you, instead of slowing you down with joint pain due to unbalanced muscle development.

Don't be surprised if you try the exercises in this book and discover soreness not only in your stomach, but in your arms, lats, chest, butt, hamstrings, and other places as well. This is what happens when you follow a full-body abdominal routine, instead of an isolated one—and it means you get better results, muscular development, and overall strength.

WARMING UP

Warming up is absolutely critical whenever you do any kind of exercise routine. It's a bad idea to go from a total rest to the stress and effort of a workout, because you can easily end up pulling or straining a muscle and injuring yourself. This is as true of ab exercises and core exercises as anything else, so make sure your muscles are always warm before you do them.

Many people do their ab routines after a normal workout routine, so by that time they have been exercising for a while and they are warm. If you are warm from the exercise you were just doing, you might be fine to move on to your ab workout. However, if you are doing this ab workout independently, or if you want to be sure your core is thoroughly warmed up, you should consider doing a few repetitions of the following warm-up exercises.

Jumping Jacks

The jumping jack is one of the most basic, well-known exercises around, and with good reason. There might not be a better, more convenient way to get your muscles working and your circulation going in your whole body than this:

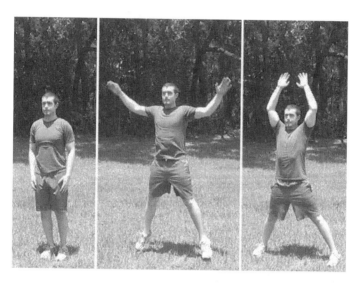

Stand with feet together and arms at your sides, then jump up and spread your legs out while lifting your arms above your head. Land with your feet spread and your arms straight up, then jump back to the starting position. A set of anywhere from 25 to 100 of these is great before this or any workout.

Trunk Twists

This is another basic if underutilized warm up exercise. This more specifically targets your entire core, so it's a good one before your ab and lower back workout.

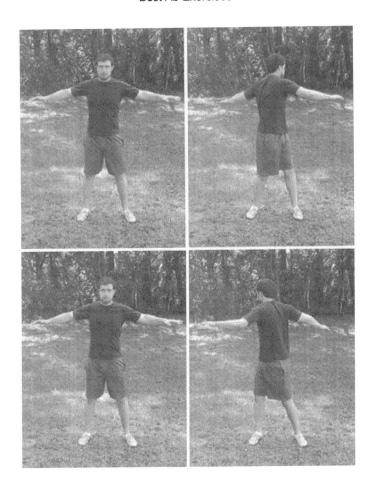

Keep your feet planted and your arms out, and be sure to twist in a smooth, controlled manner so you don't pull anything. One or two sets of 10-25 of these should be good.

*****

These warm up exercises should be all you need to prepare your entire midsection for your core workout. Get comfortable with them, and they will serve you well.

THE EXERCISES

Now that we've covered the warm up, it's time to get into the actual core exercises you'll be doing. Some of these you will have heard of, some you won't. Some will appear challenging and intimidating, some will seem pretty easy.

Regardless, I'd recommend that you approach all of them in the same way. Take the time to read about and learn each exercise, using the pictures and descriptions to be sure your form is right.

Don't underestimate the ones that might seem easy, and don't be scared of the ones that seem hard. Every one of these exercises has a place in a great overall abdominal routine, and every one of them is something you are capable of doing, even if they seem difficult at first.

Just follow the progressions as described, and you'll get there.

PLANK

This is a very popular ab exercise for the past few years, and justifiably so. It will hit your entire abdomen—and your chest and shoulders too—and it can be a great foundation for your ab exercise routine.

We'll start with the basic plank, and then look at a couple of variations to shift the focus of the exercise and/or to make it even more intense.

The basic plank is straightforward, but if you get the form wrong the effectiveness of this exercise will be greatly reduced. First, assume what is more or less a pushup position. You can hold the position with your hands on the ground, as shown, or with your forearms on the ground; either one will work.

This is the position you will hold for the entire exercise, but the position of your hips and flexion in your stomach are what really make the plank count.

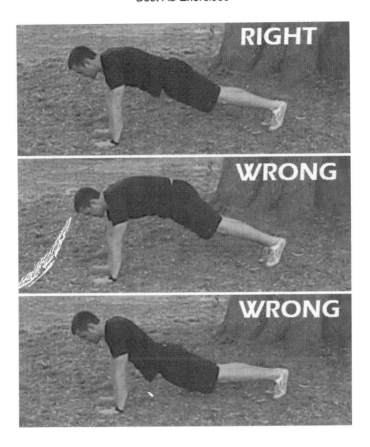

If your hips are too low, they aren't being supported by your abs, and you're not getting the ab work you need. If your hips are too high, too much support comes from your legs and shoulders, and again your abs aren't working.

You need to keep your body straight, flex your abs, and shift your hips up and down slightly until you can feel your abs working to support them, pretty much right in the middle.

Once you feel that optimal position with your abdominal muscles working to support your butt, take deep, slow breaths and flex your entire stomach hard, especially on the exhale. Hold the position for as long as you can.

Take the time to find the right position! If you're doing it right, you should really feel your abs working hard. Tweak your position as needed until you get there.

Now let's take a look at a simple variation:

Side Plank

The side plank takes the same concept as a normal plank, but shifts the target to your oblique muscles, or 'side abs.'

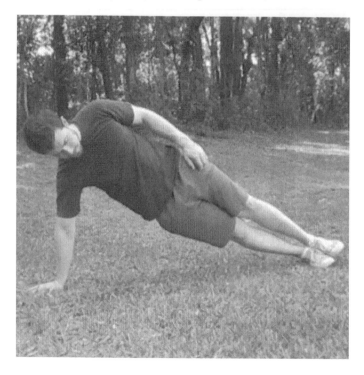

Again, this exercise can be done with your hand on the ground, or with your forearm on the ground. Pick one, and hold that position for as long as you can.

Apply the same concept from the regular plank here; you want to keep your body in a straight line, and make sure your hips are positioned in such a way that you can really feel your obliques working. The muscles that are closer to the ground are the ones you should really feel doing the work.

Once you're done with one side, switch your position and do the same amount of work on the other side. Always work both sides evenly.

Here's a cool variation that incorporates both of the previous exercises into one dynamic exercise for your chest, arms, and shoulders, as well as your abdomen:

Plank Switch

To do the plank switch, you start out in a plank position. Then, in a smooth and controlled manner, you switch to a side plank one on side with your free arm raised above you. Then, you go back to the plank. Then, switch to a side plank on the other side, and back to the plank again, and so on.

Good form counts for so much in plank exercises, and that is certainly true here. Be sure to hold each of the positions in this progression correctly, and don't rush from one to the other.

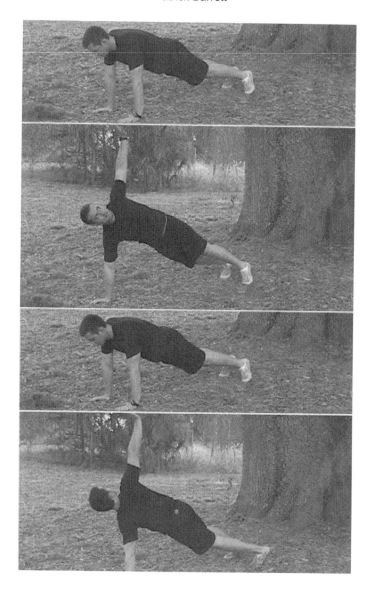

Let's check out one last variation for another option to give you a great chest, shoulder, arms, and ab workout:

Plank Push

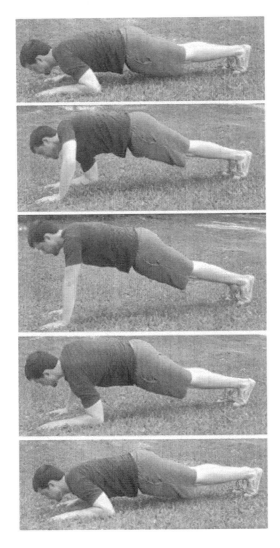

Remember for the first version of the plank, we talked about how you can do it either on your hands, or on your forearms? In this variation, you will start on your forearms. Then, you will push up onto your hands, one hand at a time. Once you are up on your hands, you will go back down on your forearms, one at a time.

One full cycle up and down is one rep.

I always like to stay balanced, so after a full cycle of going up and then down leading with one arm, I'd recommend leading with the other arm for your next full cycle of going up and down. So if you start down on both arms, and you're starting with your left, you'd go up left, up right, down left, down right, and that's one cycle. The next one would go up right, up left, down right, down left.

If that's confusing, actually do the motion yourself and pay attention to the position of each side. The order isn't crucial as long as you mirror it on both sides. Again, this might be confusing, but it will make more sense when you actually get down and do the exercise.

Notice in the pictures how my form on the forearm plank is a little off; this happens because when your drop your forearms to the ground from the pushup position, the placement isn't exactly right. The result is that one or both of your planking positions will be a little bit out of whack, but it's not something you need to worry about for this exercise.

Experiment a little bit with hand placement, keep your abs flexed, use the best form you can, and you'll get good results.

L-SIT

This is one of my favorite abdominal exercises, because it also teaches balance and body awareness and a basic gymnastic skill.

As the picture on the next page indicates, you're going to sit flat with your legs extended in front of you and press your hands into the ground to lift yourself up, so that you are supporting your full weight on your hands.

It's easier said than done, but once we look at a few details you'll be able to get there.

The first important detail is hand placement. Your hands should be placed on either side of your legs, at right around the halfway point of your femur—right in the middle between your knee and your butt. That will make sure you're starting out in the right place for optimal balance.

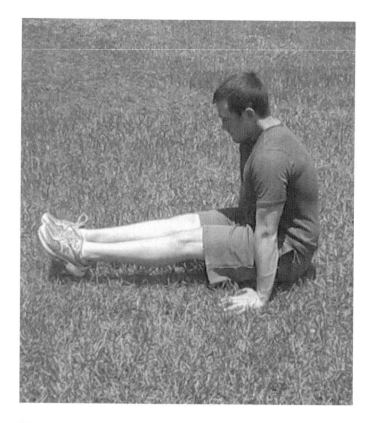

Every person's body is a little bit different, so once you get used to it you might want to come just forward or back of this placement, but it's going to be right around that area.

With your hands in place, you'll want to keep your legs extended straight, point your toes, tighten your stomach muscles, and press down on your hands. This brings us to the second important detail. In order to create enough pressure down on your hands, you'll have to consciously curl your upper abs and your shoulders downward as you press.

That will help direct the force properly so that you lift up off the ground instead of just leaning back.

In the beginning you might only be able to lift your butt off the ground, while your feet stay down, like in this picture:

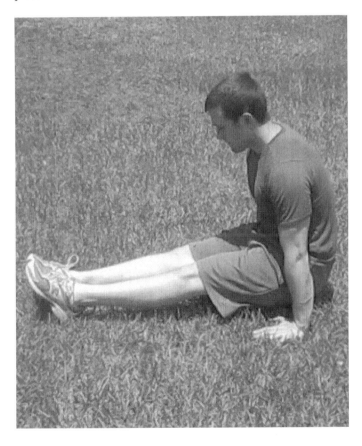

That's okay. Get used to holding that position for time, and once you get stronger, try lifting your feet up for a few seconds at a time, and progress into doing the L-sit correctly with your feet up.

Hold this position for time; keep your arms strong and straight, your lower abs tight, and your upper abs and shoulders curled down. You'll build strength in your arms, shoulders, abs, and even in your legs.

L-SIT BICYCLE

Once you've mastered the L-Sit, you can move into this variation, which will create a more intense and dynamic movement. Make sure you are fully comfortable with the first version before you get started with this one.

Essentially, you're going to start in the L-sit position. Then, you're going to lean back slightly, and draw one leg up into your chest while keeping the other straight. Then, you will straighten that leg, and draw in the other one, and so on.

You may not be able to see it clearly in the picture on the next page, but remember that the only part of your body touching the ground is your hands; your butt and legs are in the air.

In the beginning you may only be able to do this for a handful of repetitions before you fall over or just can't do it any more, but stick with it and you'll make progress.

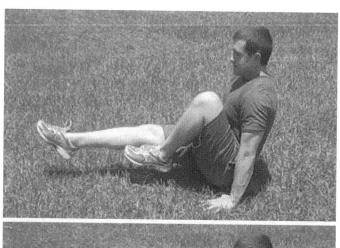

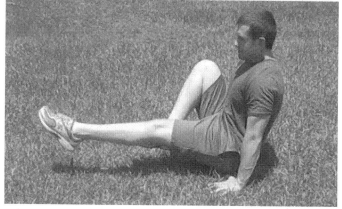

LYING LEG RAISE

There are a lot of variations on the leg raise you can use in a core workout. Unfortunately, a lot of them seem to result in discomfort in your lower back.

This version minimizes that effect, and also puts your body through a more realistic and complete range of motion.

Lie flat on the ground, with your arms extended and your hands, palms down, on the ground by your side. While pressing down with your hands for leverage, keep your legs extended as you lift them up over your head.

Continue to lift them up as far as you're comfortable lifting them, up to and including until they touch the ground behind your head. Then bring them back to their original position, and repeat. Remember to brace on the ground with your hands for leverage through the movement.

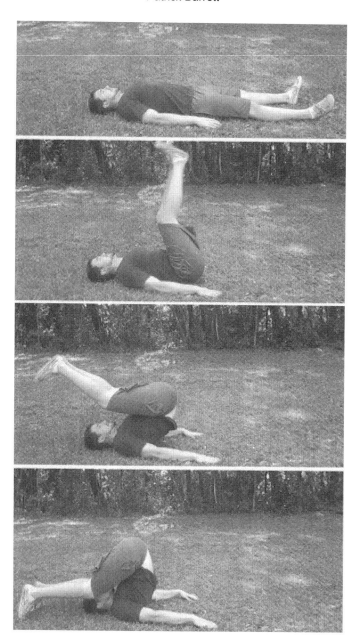

If that's a little bit challenging, there is another variation you can use.

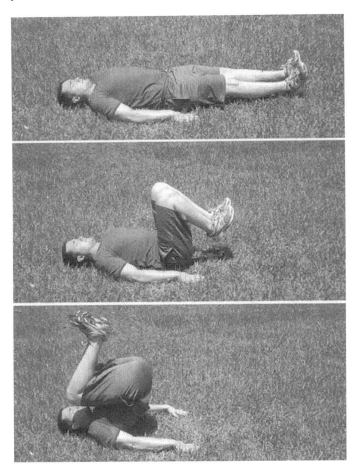

Instead of keeping your legs extended, tuck your knees up into your chest, and continue pressing with your hands as you roll your hips up off the ground. As before, continue the motion as far as you comfortably can, and then return to the original position. Again, remember to press your hands down for leverage against the weight of your legs.

Even if you can do the more difficult variation, the version where you tuck your knees is still valuable, so you might consider trading them out every other workout, or every few weeks, or just whenever you want a change. You can also alternate, doing one repetition with your legs straight, and one with your legs tucked, and so on.

HANGING LEG RAISE

This is another variation on the leg raise, and it's actually one of my favorite abdominal exercises—maybe even one of my overall favorites.

For this exercise, hang from a bar high enough that your legs are not touching the ground. Then, keeping your legs extended, lift them straight in front of you, and then all the way up so that your legs touch the bar above your head. See the picture on the next page.

Depending on your flexibility, how wide your grip on the bar is, and how long your arms and legs are, you might touch the bar with your toes, or somewhere on your shins; that's not important as long as your legs are straight and your form is good.

Once your legs are raised to about waist-high, you will need to press forward on the bar with your hands to get the leverage you need to lift your legs the rest of the way.

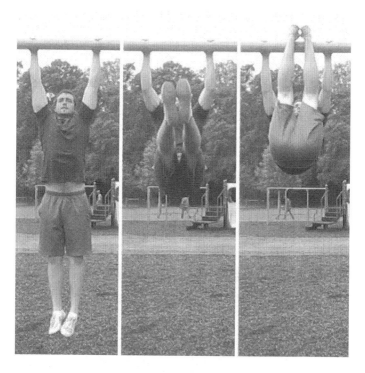

There is another variation you can do that will be slightly easier. Instead of lifting all the way, just lift your legs until they are parallel to the ground. You can start out with reps in this range, and then work your way up to the full range when you get a little stronger.

Once you can do the full motion for multiple reps, you will not only feel the workout in your abdominal muscles, but also in your lats, arms, and the backs of your shoulders.

HANGING TUCK

This is one of my favorites because it adds a decent upper body workout into a great abdominal exercise. Essentially you're going to hang from a bar, tuck your knees up into your chest, and then rotate your hips upward until your feet touch the bar to complete the range of motion.

The first part of this motion is to tuck your knees into your chest. So take a breath, and as you exhale raise your knees into this position. Then, in a fluid motion (and keeping your knees tucked), press forward with your hands and continue to lift your hips so that your body rotates backwards until the tops of your feet make contact with the bar.

Then, lower yourself in a controlled manner back through that sequence, and repeat. See the picture on the next page.

You may find this to be difficult at first. If so, start with just the first part of the motion, where you lift your knees and tuck them into your chest.

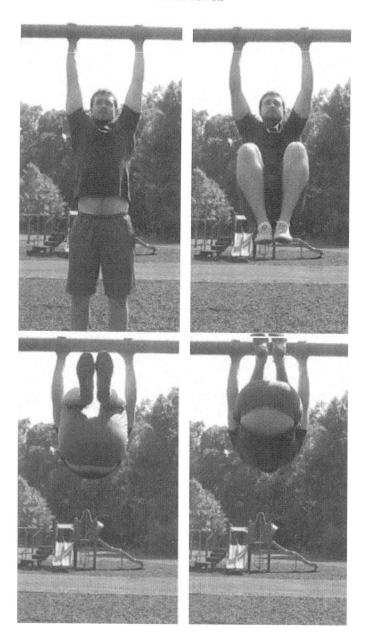

Once you are comfortable with that, get comfortable with the rotation. When you start to lift your hips, lean back a little and also push your hands forward for leverage. Just concentrate on lifting your hips upward and raising your feet toward the bar.

At first, you should only lift yourself a little bit to be sure you can safely do the exercise. As you get more sure of yourself, lift more, until you can keep rotating all the way until the tops of your feet touch the bar. Then come back down the same way.

This exercise involves hanging upside-down from the bar, so take it slow and don't do anything you aren't comfortable with. If you don't feel comfortable hanging upside down, don't do this exercise.

ARMS EXTENDED PUSHUPS

This is another great exercise for your entire abdomen as well as your chest, legs, lats, and triceps. It's pretty intense, and you definitely need to take a little time to get comfortable with it, but it's well worth the effort.

Start this exercise by lying face down on the floor. Put your toes on the ground and your hands out in front of your head with your elbows slightly bent.

Then, flex your abs and your lower back, keep your legs firmly extended, and press your hands hard into the ground. Hopefully, you'll be able to lift yourself up off the ground.

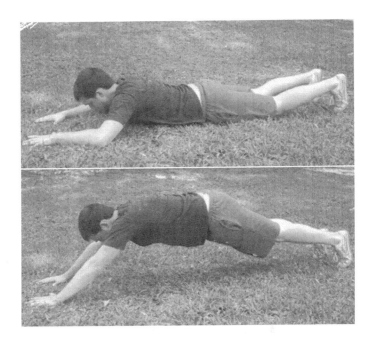

If you are unable to perform this exercise as described, you can also do the exact same thing, but plant your knees in the ground, instead of your feet.

That way is much easier, so it will give you a chance to get more comfortable with the movement in general, and it will also give you a chance to get stronger and build up to the original version of the exercise.

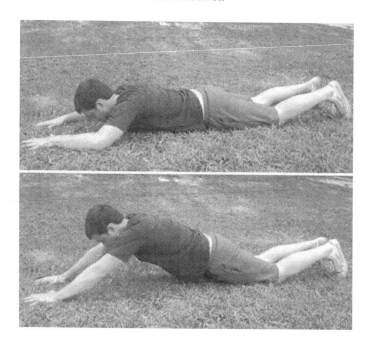

KNEE UPS

This is a great twist on a cardio-type exercise which will hit your hip flexors, obliques, and lower abs. You can do 1-3 high rep sets of these on a regular basis for great results.

Stand upright, with your hands by your sides and your feet shoulder-width apart. First bring one knee up to about chest level, then lower it, then lift the other knee to the same height, and then lower it.

Try to lift the knee as high as you comfortably can, and as you do so, kind of "crunch" that same side of your body down to meet it. Be sure to achieve a similar movement on each side of your body, and bear in mind that lifting one knee, and then the other, is one repetition.

Find a rhythm, somewhere around a walking or jogging cadence, and do high rep sets for best results. This can serve the dual purpose of doing light-to-moderate cardiovascular exercise, which will burn away the fat that

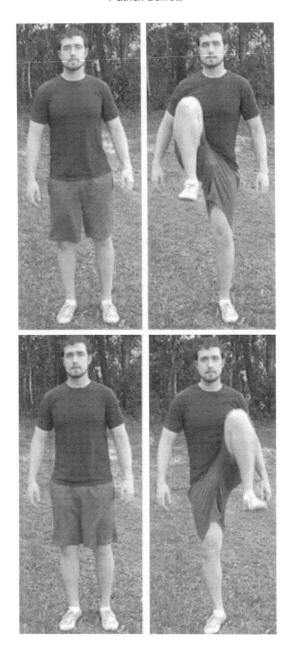

might be covering your abs, as well as light-to-moderate abdominal exercise, which will shape and tone your abs and improve their endurance.

JUMPING KNEE UPS

We're going to take the same basic concept from the last exercise and change a few things to make it significantly more intense.

For the jumping knee ups, you're going to squat down, then jump straight up into the air. On your way up, you're going to bring both knees up into your chest together, so that at the top of your jump both of them are fully tucked.

Then, straighten your legs, land, and repeat the jump until you are fatigued. See the picture on the next page.

The combination of exercising your legs along with your abs makes this a great lower body and cardiovascular workout in addition to the benefit for your hip flexors and lower abdominals. That means burning off fat and toning and strengthening your abdominals at the same time.

One quick note—you can do these with a full squat and a jump (as pictured; squat all the way down until your butt is

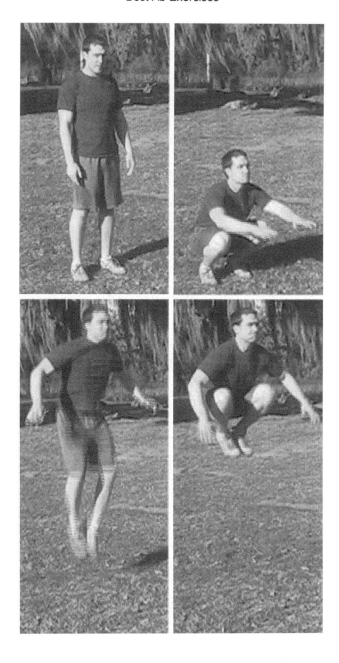

on your ankles), or you can do about a quarter-squat and a jump (squatting down a few inches with just enough bend in your legs so you can push off and perform the exercise).

The full squat jumps will obviously engage your lower body more, but you can probably do the quarter-squat jumps at a faster rate, which might raise your heart-rate more; there are benefits either way, and really whichever you prefer doing is fine.

You can also mix both into one workout, or stick with one for a few weeks, and then switch to the other for variety.

BIRDSNEST STRETCH

So many of the core exercises that you do will involve curling yourself forward into a ball in one form or another; this is a great stretch because it does the exact opposite.

For this stretch, you will begin by lying face-down on the floor. Then, reach behind yourself with one hand to grab the corresponding ankle, then with the other hand to grab the other ankle.

Once you've done this, you'll perform the stretch by lifting your shoulders, pulling forward with your hands, and extending your legs to push away from the force of your hands on your ankles.

Hold for about ten seconds or so. That will give you a great stretch in your entire abdomen, down through your hip flexors and quadriceps. See the picture on the next page for reference.

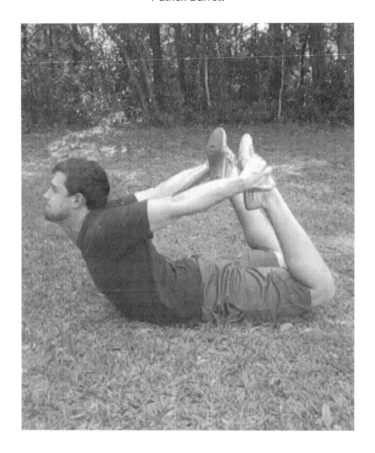

ISOMETRIC FLEXION

One of the more underappreciated abdominal exercises is isometric flexion. This is possibly the most convenient exercise there is because you can do it literally anywhere in almost any situation—at home, at work, on a bus, anywhere.

It's simple enough, although we'll look at some different aspects of the exercise and discuss some finer points.

As far as the exercise goes, all you do is inhale deeply, then exhale slowly and completely while flexing your stomach muscles.

As is the case with many exercises, attention to detail and good form will get you much greater results, so take the time to do it right!

When you're inhaling, keep your muscles flexed somewhat. But as you slowly exhale, flex them hard. The more you exhale, the more you squeeze those muscles.

Also, be sure to concentrate on flexing the top, middle, bottom, and sides of your abdomen. Consciously engage each area as you continue to exhale and squeeze. Then, release a little, inhale deeply, and repeat.

This simple exercise can do a lot for you, and can easily be modified in a number of ways. Let's look at a few of those.

Seated Ab Flexion

This is pretty self-explanatory, but I just want to call attention to the versatility of the exercise.

As the name implies, you can do this exercise while sitting down—though you should do your best to maintain good posture while doing so (and in general) for best results.

Think about that—you can do ab exercises while riding in a car or on a bus, while in class or in a meeting, while you watch TV or a movie. You can do it almost anywhere, and it really works. So use it.

Standing Ab Flexion

Along the same lines we were just talking about, you can also do this while standing in a lot of different situations. You can be waiting in line, standing on the subway, or doing almost anything, and you can be working on your breathing, posture, and abdominal development at the same time.

Hanging Ab Flexion

This gets a little more interesting, if a little less convenient. This exercise can also be done while hanging from a bar—stretching your body out in this way will put you abdomen in a slightly different position, and variety is almost always a good thing in your exercise routine.

It also throws in the variable of hanging by your hands, which means your upper body, particularly your hands and forearms, is also engaged. Just get on the bar, hang still, and follow the same inhaling, then exhaling and flexing pattern we discussed earlier.

Walking Ab Flexion

You don't need to be still to get the benefits of isometric ab flexion. Performing this exercise while your legs are moving back and forth adds another great dimension to this exercise.

It also takes walking—which is a great daily habit to get into—and makes it into a much more significant fat-burning event without adding any more time. Walking is great because it means getting fresh air and promoting circulation, which is vital to your good health, and it heightens both of those components by making the breathing deeper and more intense, and also adds in a core workout.

If you only take a few things away from this book, this section on isometric flexion needs to be one of them. People complain about not having enough time to exercise; we've now discussed several ways that you can do this exercise while you're doing something else—without going to the gym, without changing your clothes, without people around you even realizing that you're working out.

This is great information, so be sure you make use of it!

LOWER BACK EXERCISES

These last two exercises primarily target your lower back, a very important part of your body which many people ignore. This is an especially serious mistake when you spend a lot of time working out your stomach and do nothing to exercise the complementary muscles in your lower back.

It is no coincidence that many people also suffer through bad posture and lower back pain as they get older, so we want to be sure to include this type of exercise in our workouts.

While many exercises incorporate your lower back (in the same way that many incorporate your abdominal muscles), it's good to have a few regular ones like these that target it more directly. Using these in your routine regularly will help to balance out all of the stomach work you're doing by developing a strong, healthy, pain-free lower back.

Let's take a look.

SUPERMAN

This is a great exercise for an often-neglected part of your core—your lower back.

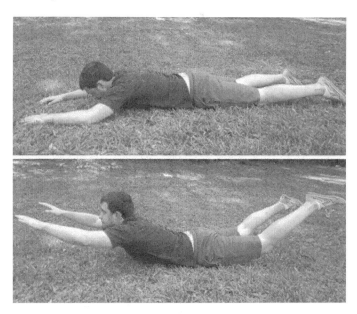

Just lie flat on the ground on your stomach, with your legs straight and your your hands palms-down on the floor in front of your head. Then, keeping your arms and legs relatively straight, lift your legs, as well as your arms and chest, up off the ground.

You can hold the up position for time, and you can also do repetitions. This will focus on your lower back but also work out your upper back, shoulders, butt, and hamstrings.

If that's a little too challenging, there's another variation that might be a bit easier.

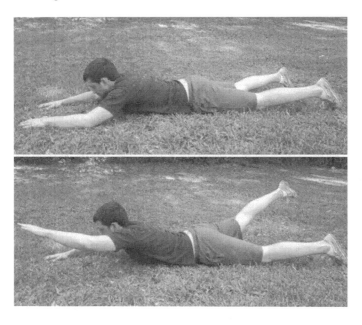

In this variation, instead of lifting both arms and legs simultaneously, alternate lifting opposite arms and legs—for example, lift your left arm and right leg, then lower them and lift you right arm and left leg, and so on. When you lift one arm and leg, use the lowered ones to brace against the ground for leverage.

Once you get pretty good at this version, you can move up to the regular version where you lift both legs and your chest and arms all together.

WRESTLER'S BRIDGE

If you've read my other books, you might know by now that anytime I write about a full body or core workout I have to include the wrestler's bridge. Even though it doesn't directly work out your abdominal muscles, it might be the best exercise out there for your lower back, and I think it's probably the best single all-around exercise there is, since it incorporates your neck, shoulders, and lower body as well.

You may not be familiar with this exercise, and if you aren't, it might appear to be strange and intimidating. Don't worry. We're going to walk through it step-by-step.

There are two different versions we're going to look at. The first one is a little easier and will be better for beginners, and the second one is actually a correct wrestler's bridge. Let's take a look at the first one.

Bridge Part 1

It's a little difficult to describe without visual aids, so let's start by looking at some pictures.

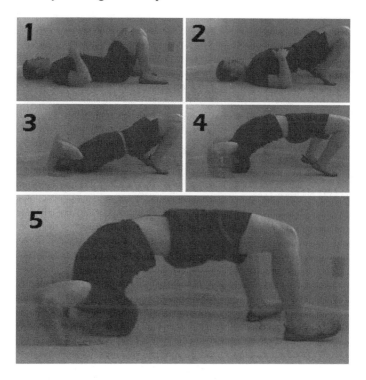

As you can see, you're going to lie down on your back, and then bring your heels up near your butt.

Then, scoot yourself toward your feet a little bit until your butt is up off the ground a little and your weight is on your feet and your head and shoulders.

Next, plant your hands on the ground on either side of your head, lift up your head, and then place the top of your head on the ground so that your weight is on your feet, head, and hands.

In this position, try to thrust your hips upward so that your body makes a sort of upside-down "U." Also, as much as you're comfortable, try to roll slowly forward so that your weight moves from the top of your head to your forehead, and even to your nose. These two actions will help provide the lion's share of the benefit in simultaneously strengthening and stretching your lower back, upper back, and neck.

Now let's look at the next version, which is really a correct wrestler's bridge.

Bridge Part 2

This is very similar to the last version we looked at, except now you will do the last part without any support from your hands.

As you work on the first version of the bridge (using your hands for support), you want your goal to be to hold that position with more and more of your weight supported by your head, and less and less weight supported by your hands. Do this simply by consciously pressing down with your hands less so that your head must pick up the slack.

When you've done the first version a few times and you start to feel comfortable, try slowly lifting your hands up off the ground. If you're able to do that, then cross your arms over your chest and hold that position for as long you feel comfortable doing it.

You may have gotten used to doing the easier version of the bridge with your weight on your forehead or even down by your nose. Even if you can do that with your hands on the ground, the first time you lift your hands up you may want to have your weight closer to the top of your head, because you might feel stronger there.

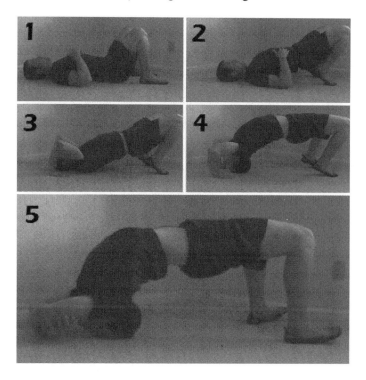

Your goal later on is still to get your weight forward onto your forehead and then onto your nose, but for now just focus on doing what you need to do to hold the bridge without your hands on the ground.

Even if in the beginning you can only hold it for a few seconds, that's still great because you're getting started. From there, get comfortable holding it for five or ten seconds, then 20 or 30 seconds, then a minute or more.

As you increase the time for which you can hold the bridge, you also want to continue to flex your butt and thrust your hips up more and roll farther forward on your head. If you can bridge up to your nose, and hold that for two to three minutes or more, you're doing very well.

Again, I know this is an unusual exercise, but take your time, take it step by step, and only move forward when you're comfortable. You'll be surprised what you can do.

MAKE IT A PART OF YOUR WORKOUT

So now you know a full set of ab exercises. The next topic we need to address is how to fit those into your exercise routine.

There are a lot of ways to do this, but we'll cover the most important aspect of this topic first: balance.

Most people focus on the idea of ab exercises, or developing a six pack, or something else along those lines. However, you must take care to exercise your lower back as well for the sake of balance.

To put it simply, your stomach muscles and back muscles work together in a lot of common movements, and if one of the two groups is much more developed than the other group, you increase the likelihood of injury, bad posture, back pain, and other problems.

It's not necessarily accurate to say you have to spend exactly the same amount of time on each one, only that you should take care to get in a great lower back workout roughly as often as you get a great ab workout.

There are probably a whole lot more ab-focused exercises out there than there are lower back-focused exercises, and that certainly holds true in this book. But, there are still two great exercises you've learned that primarily target your lower back—the wrestler's bridge and the superman.

As I said before, I really think the wrestler's bridge is one of the best exercises out there—probably the best, actually. I like to do it once a day, for as long as I can comfortably hold it, around 5-7 times a week.

That alone will give you great strength in your lower back, but the superman (either version, or both) is also a great exercise that you should incorporate into your regular workout routine.

The other type of balance, which is also very important but a little more obvious, is left-to-right balance. Basically, if you spend a certain amount of time planking on one side, you should spend the same amount on the other side, and you should keep reps and sets and time even on both sides when an exercise does each side individually, and so on.

Some of you have a well-developed sense of how to build a workout routine. If you feel comfortable and confident that you know how to do that already, then go for it.

Here's an explanation for those of you who don't:

First, bear in mind the balance we talked about just now. Most of this is ab stuff, but don't forget to do the exercises for your lower back too.

Second, pick some exercises. You can do all the exercises in this book, or you can pick a few that look interesting to you, and incorporate the others later (be sure to give them all a shot though, so you don't miss a potential favorite).

Next, figure out when to do them.

To keep things straightforward, we'll break these exercises up into two major groups: exercises you can do for ten or more reps at a time, and exercises you can't do ten reps at a time.

If you can't do 10 reps of a certain ab exercise in good form, you should treat it like you would most other difficult bodyweight exercises. Do 3-5 sets of maybe 4-8 reps (whatever you can do) around 2-4 times a week, with a minute or two of rest between sets.

These exercises are more difficult, so you need to do more sets to get in more reps (since you can't do many reps at a time) and you need at least a full day of recovery after your workout in most cases. They will help to build real abdominal strength and will also probably increase the size of your abdominal muscles.

The other exercises will be easier; you can hold them for a long time, or you can do them for a lot of reps (more than 10, anyway). You should do 1-3 higher-rep sets of these exercises 4-6 times a week. Because they are less strenuous, you need to do more of them, more often to feel the benefits, but in return they will help you to build lean, toned abdominal muscles.

I always like to point out that a decent workout routine that you follow is infinitely better than a perfect routine that you don't follow. With that in mind, be aware that these are not hard and fast rules, but general guidelines. If you need to tweak these a little bit to create a workout that you can follow, that's no problem at all; as long as it's a challenge and you stick with it and don't hurt yourself, you should be fine.

When it comes to figuring out an ab routine, most people will probably just pick a handful of exercises they like and do them all in a row three, or four, or five times a week.

That's completely fine. I just want to lay this out so you don't get mixed up when you find that some exercises seem a little too easy or a little too hard; different exercises will require different recovery times, and you might want to make some adjustments with certain exercises to account for that.

Perhaps the best approach for this routine is to do super sets. Here's an explanation if you don't know what that means.

Let's say you're doing three exercises, to keep it easy. Instead of doing one set of exercise 1, then resting, then another set, then resting, and so on until you're done with that exercise, and then moving on to exercise 2, and so on, doing "super sets" means you would do a set of exercise 1, then a set of exercise 2, then a set of exercise 3, then another set of exercise 1, then 2, then 3, and so on until you are done, with little or no rest in between. That way you spend less time resting and more time working, and your workout takes less time.

To make that a little more concrete, we'll pick three basic sample exercises: the plank, the lying leg lift, and the superman. In this example, you might do:

Plank: 30 seconds

Lying leg lift: 10 repetitions

Superman: 15 repetitions

You would do those three exercises right in a row, and start back on the first exercise (the plank) as soon as you finished the last one (superman). You would also do the whole series through 3-5 times to complete your abdominal workout.

Now, bear in mind that this is only a sample. It may be on the easy side for some people, and you might want to choose more exercises once you feel comfortable with them—maybe more like 4-6 to do in a series.

This approach—super setting the exercises all in a row, instead of doing each one with rest in between—takes a lot less time and is, obviously, a lot more intense. It will also get you better results in less time.

Because it is intense, though, you should ease into it; always take baby steps so that you know you are physically ready for whatever you're going to do. Start with fewer exercises, fewer sets, fewer reps, and once you're comfortable you should build up until you're getting a good workout.

When you start doing a new set of exercises, your body will usually respond positively, and you will find them to be challenging. But your body will adapt, and you will get stronger and better at them.

You've got to adapt too, and keep challenging yourself. Try different variations. Increase the reps and sets. Every few weeks, drop a few exercises, and add a few new ones. Later on, mix the exercises up again.

When you exercise for strength and health, whether or not you're focusing on your abdomen, long-term success depends on variety over time and continuing to challenge yourself. Stay on top of things. When you get stronger and this gets easier, find new ways to make yourself work hard.

HOW ELSE CAN YOU WORK YOUR CORE?

This book covers many different ways that you can exercise your entire abdomen as well as your lower back. Many of these exercises also hit other areas of your body.

That's only logical, because your body is built to work as a unit. Many people like to isolate one muscle group or another when they work out, especially when their goals have more to do with appearance and less to do with strength.

This can result in overdeveloped muscles in one area, and underdeveloped muscles in another area—and when those two muscle groups try to work together, you can strain something and injure yourself.

Anyway, just as the exercises contained in this book work out more than just your core, a good workout for the rest of your body should also give your core a workout. In fact, many good exercises will engage your core on some level:

—Pushups, in good form, can be a great ab exercise (after all, you're holding a plank the whole time).

—Pullups can also hit your abs.

—Squats will exercise your lower back.

—Many sports will give you a great core workout, because they take place in a dynamic environment and your core must work so it can create stability for your body while you play.

You can see the pattern here. It's important that you not look at the exercises in this book, or at other ab exercises, and think they are the only ones that work your core.

As you do other exercises, take the time to notice the role that your abs and lower back play in whatever you're doing. Consciously noticing how those muscles are helping out in whatever you're doing gives you a chance to get them more actively involved, which has the double benefit of both improving that motion and further strengthening your core.

BUILDING THE ABS YOU WANT

Core exercise is very important if you want to be as strong as possible. You can't really do anything that requires real strength if your body itself is not stable, and it is your abdominal muscles and lower back that provide the bulk of that stability.

It follows from that that the stronger you want to be, the more you have to make sure your core strength keeps up with the rest of your body so the power you're developing translates to use in the real world.

Having said all of that, the primary reason that most people focus on exercising their abdomen is so it looks better. While I always like to advocate that your first goal should be your health and strength, and your second goal be an improved appearance, I can certainly understand the desire to have a nicer looking stomach as opposed to a fleshy gut with no muscle tone.

With that in mind, we should get a few things straight. There are a number of things that you can do which will have an impact on the appearance of your stomach and your abdominal muscles, and it's worth it to go through those one by one so you can decide on the best course of action for you.

Heavy Ab Exercise

When you work out your biceps, or your chest, or your butt, you expect them to get bigger, right? Well, the same thing happens when you work out your abdominal muscles. Although many people have the goal of decreasing their waistlines, few realize that intense ab exercise actually often increases the size of your stomach area, to an extent, simply by developing and enlarging your ab muscles.

We are talking here about more intense ab exercise—kind of like when you target another muscle group and you hit it hard just a few times a week and give it a few days to recover. You'll build strength as well as size.

At the same time, exercise will help to burn fat, so if you're exercising enough you will also lose the fat covering those muscles, and you will start to develop the lean stomach with visible abs that many people are looking for—so the muscles might get bigger, but the fat over them gets smaller for an overall decrease in stomach size.

Of course, all of that depends on where you're starting from, how developed your abs are already, and how much weight you've got to lose. Let's take a look at the next situation.

Light Ab Exercise

This category has more to do with a higher repetition routine that you would do almost every day. In this case, the ab muscles are developed, but they gain more in tone and less in size. This falls in line with what most people are probably looking for when they do an ab routine—more visible and developed abdominal muscles.

Bear in mind, though, that this approach might contribute less to the overall real world strength that you acquire through your ab training, since the training itself is less strenuous.

Let's look at the last type of exercise:

Non-Ab Exercise

Surprisingly enough, one behavior that has a huge impact on the appearance of your midsection is the exercise you do that doesn't target your midsection.

Yes, this is true in part because almost any good exercise you do should in some way engage your core, and that will help develop those muscles, but that isn't what I'm talking about.

For most people, it's all the other exercise they do that really determines the size of their midsections—because whether they are runners, weightlifters, athletes, fitness-class-goers, or whatever else, it's all that extra activity that actually burns the fat and keeps it from covering up their abs.

Keep this in mind—even if your main goal is "just to have a nice-looking stomach," you should still work to reap the benefits of a full-body workout.

Now let's take a look at the last component of this formula:

Diet

The food you eat has a huge impact on the appearance of your stomach. If you're serious about making a change in this department, then your diet will come into play.

Unfortunately, many sources are way off base in this department, and if you'd like to learn about a different way to understand the human diet, you might want to take a look at my book on the subject, The Natural Diet. It's a focused, easy-to-understand explanation of what's best for your body, and it will teach you how to eat a natural diet that's actually convenient and affordable as well as delicious and filling.

It's a great book for anyone who has felt confused by all the diet advice out there and wants something that works, is concrete, and just makes sense, and if that sounds interesting to you then I'd recommend you check it out. However, for the purposes of this section, we'll review some of the ideas in there that are directly related to the idea of losing weight.

This is something you could easily go on and on about, but to keep it simple I've condensed it into four main pieces of advice.

1. Reduce or Eliminate Consumption Of Processed Carbohydrates

The best way to add fat to your body is to start eating a lot of bread, pasta, potatoes, corn syrup, and similar foods.

Conversely, one of the best ways to reverse that process is to eliminate or severely limit your intake of such foods.

Many people are adjusted to the attitude that it's "normal" to snack on crackers, pretzels, chips, or other such foods during the day, or to have them as a side item with your lunch. Similarly, we think that almost any cooked meal should include potatoes or pasta. None of these are necessary, and all are adding to your waistline.

These foods generally contain little in terms of valuable nutrients, and they are quickly stored as fat. I won't tell you that you can't ever have them and be healthy—obviously that's not true. But I wouldn't recommend that any of these foods be a part of your daily routine.

This leads well into the next piece of advice.

2. Eat Fresh Fruit

If you aren't eating any of those processed carbohydrates, where are those sugars that your body needs going to come from?

Well, luckily for us fresh fruit is perhaps the most perfect food out there for your body. It's extremely easy for your body to digest, it's packed with vitamins and minerals, and it's an energy source that the human body has been using quite effectively for millenia.

Be careful here—fresh must mean fresh. Simply being made from fruit, or even containing 100% fruit, doesn't cut it. We are not talking about pasteurized fruit juice, or chopped fruit in a can. It must be real, actual, recognizable fruit from the produce section, or a farmer's market, or wherever.

If you're eating anything else that is just fruit-derived, all bets are off. Stick with fresh fruit, and make it a large part of your diet every day.

3. Avoid UNNATURAL Fats

It might seem counter-intuitive, but even though you want to lose fat from your body, eating fat is still important—you just need to eat the right fats.

Many people are familiar with the idea that there are good fats and bad fats out there. Unfortunately, most of those people are a little mixed up on which ones are good and which ones are bad.

As with fruit, you want to eat fats that are natural and unprocessed. The bad news is that most of the fats out there in most foods, and most kitchens, are highly processed and damaged. In fact, they are so processed and damaged that they smell awful, and they have to be deodorized before they can even be sold.

So since we have limited space to discuss this topic in full, that's the rule of thumb we'll use. Use fats that still have the odor and the flavor of what they came from. Soy oil (a.k.a. vegetable oil) and canola oil are out—just open the bottle and smell them. They are highly processed and introduce a lot of unnatural stuff into your body. They are also deodorized, which leaves them with no flavor or odor.

On the other hand, olive oil, peanut oil, coconut oil, palm oil, and yes, even butter, are good news. These are fats that are very close to their natural state and still have that appealing odor and aroma (that's your body telling you that you should eat something, by the way).

People tend to spend their time worrying about whether fats are saturated or unsaturated, but I would recommend that you worry about whether they are natural or unnatural. Avoid fats with no flavor or odor, avoid "spreads" with a dozen different ingredients, and stick with fats that your body can actually smell and taste.

4. Drink Water

When scientists analyze other planets to find out if they can support life, do they scour the surface for traces of diet soda?

No.

They look for water, because water is the single most important substance needed to sustain life as we know it. So many processes in your body depend on the presence of water. That includes the ones that allow your body to use up the fuel (fat) that it has stored.

You need to drink water regularly, and the water in a soda can doesn't count. In fact, unless you're freshly juicing your own fruit, or drinking organic whole milk, or having freshly brewed green tea, water should probably be the only thing you're drinking.

This serves two purposes—one is that most of the non-water drinks out there are full of either corn syrup or artificial sweeteners (both terrible for you). They are highly processed and unhealthy.

The other purpose is that as important as it is to avoid those drinks, it's even more important that your body have a regular supply of fresh water. So drink it.

*****

There's more to say about human nutrition, and if you want a more complete explanation, take a look at my book, The Natural Diet. However, you can also just stick with these tips and see great results.

So, now we've looked at four different things that impact the strength and appearance of your stomach: heavy ab exercise, light ab exercise, non-ab exercise, and diet. Each one plays a role in how your stomach looks and what it is able to do in the real world. So what's the perfect formula?

Probably unsurprisingly, you should be aware of and use all of these components in your workout—the heavier, more intense ab exercises that you can't do for very long, the lighter exercises, the unrelated exercise, and a healthy diet. All of these things combined will work together to give you the best results in the least time.

I do want to point out again that I don't normally spend this amount of time talking about how an exercise will impact your appearance. That's not my priority when I exercise and I don't think it should be yours; strength and health should come first and an attractive physique will follow.

However, this is a book about ab exercises, and most people who read it will probably have the goal of developing a more attractive, flatter midsection. There are a lot of factors that play a role in that, and I didn't want anybody to be confused about why, after doing only hanging leg lifts, their enlarged abdominal muscles were actually making their stomachs look bigger and not leaner, or anything else along those lines.

So the answer is, as it always seems to be, to do a balanced assortment of different exercises, and to eat right and work out your whole body. Who saw that coming?

CONCLUSION

When you hear people talking about working out their abs, they are most often doing it for cosmetic reasons. That's very common, and it's totally fine, and if that is your goal, then you can certainly use these exercises successfully to do that.

However, there is also a very real opportunity here to provide the "missing piece," so to speak, and possibly make yourself much stronger and fitter, too. A strong core creates more stability throughout your entire body, and when you introduce that stability into many real world situations (sports, physical labor, etc.), you may notice a big change.

This is especially true if you develop your core through exercises, like the ones in this book, that focus on your abs or lower back but also incorporate other major muscle groups in your body. You train in a way that bridges your core strength to the rest of your body, so you're ready to do the same thing out in the real world.

If you are an athlete, and you make good use of these exercises along with your overall workout routine, you could see a dramatic difference. Even if you're not, you can certainly achieve the "abdominal makeover" that many people are looking for by understanding and following the advice in this book.

But none of that will happen if you don't actually do the exercises. Owning the book is a good first step. Reading it is even better. But the only way any of that will actually make a difference is if you take what you learn and actually start doing it, and keep doing it, on a regular basis.

When you see people who are in great shape, they aren't the ones who know the newest workouts, or who do secret exercises that no one else knows. They're just people who regularly work at their fitness goals. So get out there and put this stuff to use, and you'll be very happy with the results.

ABOUT THE AUTHOR

Patrick Barrett has been interested in exercise ever since he started to lift weights with his dad and older brothers as a kid. He participated in a half-dozen organized sports (most notably inline hockey and high school wrestling) until a neck injury during a wrestling match in his junior year prevented him from playing further in any contact sports.

After the injury, he developed an interest in pursuing strength and balance, particularly through bodyweight and self-taught gymnastic-type exercises.

Patrick has always loved both cooking and eating food. Unsatisfied with the confusing and often contradictory nutritional advice offered by mainstream sources, Patrick searched for another way to understand human nutrition that was logical, consistent, and effective. His books on food and nutrition reflect this 'cleaner,' more intuitive and useful understanding of food and how it impacts our health.

Patrick hopes that his books will save his audience time and aggravation by finally offering practical ways to achieve their nutrition and fitness goals.

OTHER BOOKS BY PATRICK BARRETT

Natural Exercise: *Basic Bodyweight Training and Calisthenics for Strength and Weight-Loss*

Advanced Bodyweight Exercises: *An Intense Full Body Workout In A Home Or Gym*

The Natural Diet: *Simple Nutritional Advice For Optimal Health In The Modern World*

How To Do A Handstand: *From the Basic Exercises To The Free Standing Handstand Pushup*

Easy Exercises: *Simple Workout Routine For Busy People In The Office, At Home, Or On The Road*

Hand And Forearm Exercises: *Grip Strength Workout And Training Routine*

One Arm Pull Up: *Bodyweight Training And Exercise Program For One Arm Pull Ups And Chin Ups*

Made in the USA
Lexington, KY
18 October 2013